Confessions
of an
OPERATING ROOM
NURSE
FIFTY SHADES OF GREEN

KATE RICHARDSON, RN CPN(C)

Dedication:

This book is dedicated to

Mike
Kris
Grant
and operating room nurses everywhere
(now known as perioperative nurses)

Special thanks to several of my colleagues for their
inspirations, ideas and constant encouragement.
Extra special thanks to my son Kris for his hours of
computer help and never ending patience.

Original illustrations by D. Babishuk RN BScN CPN(C)
Final illustrations by Leo Latte
Rough editing by Tamara Shifman
Final editing by Emily, Grant and Corinne

ONE FOOT NOTE "WHO CAN KEEP THEIR HEAD"
FROM THE POEM "IF" BY RUDYARD KIPLING

Table of Contents

Preface

For many years (forty-two, actually!) I have wanted to share with other nurses—and anyone who would like to know—what an operating room nurse *really* does. It is my attempt to explain, with humor, the vast role we play and the incredible skill set we possess. Sometimes, health professionals who work in other specialty areas, and the general public, need a tiny eye opener about life in the operating room. It seems so foreign to those outside the industry. Patients want to forget the operating room, which can make OR nurses feel rather like the dentist: some poor bloke that no one wants to visit. But we really are people, too. We are fun loving; we are mothers, fathers, wives, husbands…the whole ball of wax! Yes, we are hurried and harried, but we try very hard to individualize the needs of each patient. We know you are scared! So, relax now and catch a glimpse into our world.

Enjoy!

ODE TO THE OR NURSE

Who has the bladder of an elephant and is able to stand still in stressful situations for eight hours?

Who has the eyes of an eagle and can find tiny lost needles on terrazzo floors?

Who is able to leap over tangles of extension cords, cautery cords, light sources, and drill cables with grace?

An OR nurse, that's who!

Who has hair flatter than a seal and hands dryer than sandpaper?

Who can keep her head when those around her are losing theirs and blaming it on her?

Who can calculate doses, mix drugs and yet drop it all to catch a flailing patient?

An OR nurse, that's who!

Who can never dress down on Fridays because she's always dressed down?

Who can run for a desperately needed instrument, speed back, and slide through the door, only to be told, "I don't need it now"?

Who can organize, traumatize, and agonize to keep the day on time but, alas, the best laid plans…

An OR nurse, that's who!

Who can last all day with no lunch and wear an apron of lead, a mask, a visor, a gown, and gloves with no air-conditioning, and not complain too much?

An OR nurse, that's who!

Who can navigate ten pans of high-tech instruments and see one crucial piece missing?

Who refrains from violence when someone asks, "Oh, do you just hand instruments to a doctor?"

An OR nurse, that's who!

Who puts the Count from *Sesame Street* to shame by counting to five more times in a day than even *he* can imagine?

Who accommodates so a surgeon or anesthesiologist can finish the day early, only to be rewarded with another emergency case?

Who knows the difference between an *uvulopatalopharyngoplasty* and an *esophagogastrectomy*

An OR nurse, that's who!

Who can write faster than a speeding bullet while still listening to every word a surgeon says?

Who can maintain the ever-changing standards of care, yet still be unfortunately involved in legal issues?

Who can keep cool in the face of emergencies hour after hour and not lose it?

An OR nurse, that's who!

Who runs to the cupboard to fetch supplies but the cupboard is bare?

Who calls Central Supply to beg for a special tool, only to be told, "You already have it." I don't think so!

Who answers phones, pagers, bellboys, iPhones, and Blackberries plus takes pictures and videos, and *really* wants to say, "Would you like fries with that?"

An OR nurse, that's who!

Who has her coffee break at ten forty-five and her lunch break at eleven fifteen? Yikes, it's hard to diet!

Who listens to loud music and whining surgeons and at the same time does reams of charting? Talk about multitasking,

Who works Christmas, Easter, and summer and is made to feel she's lucky to get a day off?

You guessed it—an OR nurse, that's who!

Introduction

NOW YOU ARE READY TO BEGIN!

An OR nurse is a trained registered nurse with a post-graduate operating room course and an extra designation as a "certified" peri-operative nurse (one more exam).

The OR course varies from province to province and state to state. It is taken at a community college and typically 6 months in length.

The certification is a national credential acquired through an exam and continuing learning and professional development to maintain competence. It requires recertification every 5 years.

There are other certifications which include CPR and Laser courses.

"But what is OR nursing?" you may ask. "Is it just handing instruments to the surgeon?"

Actually, that may only be one-one hundredth of the role!

OR nursing is like no other type of nursing. It has it all and then some!

- It involves patient contact—when a patient is at their most vulnerable and afraid.

- It involves daily change, accompanied by ample stress.

- It is high-tech with computer-driven equipment, monitors of every description, lasers of many types, countless machines to learn, drills, saws, pneumatic tourniquets, laparoscopic tools, and staplers for everything!

- It involves high stress and pressure, working side by side with surgeons and anesthesiologists, and two other nurses, and on a *good* day, another half nurse!

- It is high speed all day long. Time is of the essence, as we are against the clock every minute. If we fall behind by just a few minutes, the last patient runs the risk of being canceled. So our efficiency is very important.

- It is a highly skilled job on every level, from administering a myriad of drugs and mixtures, narcotics, and blood and blood products to operating cell saver equipment.

- It is choosing from a multitude of prostheses: hip, knee, eye, shoulder, and breast with *no* room for error.

- It is the epitome of teamwork! Unlike many areas of medicine, the OR nurses require a team to complete the many different types of intricate surgery, from replacing the lens in an eye to transplanting a kidney or a lung. OR nurses never work alone, unlike nurses who work in other areas of the hospital.

- It is working under a microscope to reattach limbs, make a new breast for cancer patients, or replace hips and discs in the back.

- It is not for the faint of heart! It can be gruesome and very dirty. Emergencies can happen at any time.

- It is dangerous, with the risk of being cut by the many needles and scalpel blades, saws, or wires that are used, obviously some tainted with HIV Aids or Hepatitis C.

- It is heavy work, since our patients are all asleep and must be lifted. Limbs must be held. The instrument pans weigh more than twenty pounds, and we may have to lift ten of these several times for just one type of surgery!

All in all, it is not just handling instruments but instead requires a whole host of skills.

Despite it all, we love what we do and wouldn't work anywhere else. There is always room for fun and jokes but, alas, no time for "lunch and learns"! The medical staff has tremendous trust in their nurses, but this adds pressure to have everything available and in good working order. At the end of the day, there is always special thanks and praise for a job well done.

CHAPTER 1

A Day in the Life

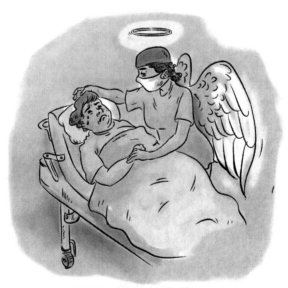

The Comforting Angel of Mercy

Does an OR nurse just hand instruments?

Well, I think you get the picture—definitely not! Preparation for a full day of surgery begins the day before. The nurse in charge of each particular operating room must choose the instruments and equipment needed for each case. Usually these are ordered through a computer program.

Early in the morning, before birds and most people are up, the OR nurse hustles around arranging for the day. In our hospital, we are exceptionally busy so we have a full night shift. These ladies of the night see to it that the day shift has the many pieces of equipment needed to start the first case of the day in each of the nine operating rooms. At the same time, they are also tackling the emergency cases. Talk about multitasking! Some hospitals have twenty-five rooms—imagine the work to set those up plus deal with emergencies!

Remember your friend who had to have an emergency Caesarean section to save her baby…or herself? That's the job of your OR nurse who has just spent several hours setting up cases and perhaps helped put a patient with stab wounds back together or reattached a finger. It's usually about four a.m. when babies want to come into the world, and they wait for no one.

Finally, at seven-thirty a.m., the day nurses arrive. We proceed to various room assignments, hoping not too many staff members have called in sick. You see, when someone from the OR calls in sick, replacements cannot be found from the hospital pool because it is too specialized an area. We either run short or pray a part-timer can be found on short notice.

Every OR is different. Some rooms have many short cases, necessitating a quick changeover, while others have very long cases, requiring tons of fancy equipment.

As the day starts to unfold, the rest of the team gathers. This often includes respiratory technologists, surgical assists, X-ray technicians, sales reps, and in big teaching hospitals, interns, residents, fellows, and of course, the surgeon and anesthesiologist. When all are present, including the patient, we complete our "Surgical Safety Checklist" after bringing the patient into the room.

Now the day has begun, and each case begins in the same manner: praying that no nurse is ill or has to leave because his or her child is sick. In the event that one nurse has to go home, there are precious few replacements, and now you are left with no one to let you go to lunch. This is unfortunate, as we nurses really like to eat! This necessitates what we call "breaking," which simply means we finish one surgery and then go to lunch—thereby delaying the next person and, of course, all subsequent patients.

However, we first have to grovel with the surgeon, who doesn't want to delay his or her day, and then usually listen to the whining for the rest of the day for allowing us our thirty minutes of unpaid lunch—that's right. We don't get paid for lunch. Lunch and learn? Not us! Our patients come first. The rest of the hospital may think we like to hide away in the OR, but in fact, it's the nature of the job. This is the same reason we are rarely able to go to the cafeteria. There's just no time. This is another reason why we become so close-knit—we don't get out much!

Every case is so different—the surgeon is different, the patient is different, and the challenge is adjusting to the many changes. Many pieces of the puzzle must fit together to make it all happen. This is what we OR nurses thrive on: the fast pace, the technical challenges, and the ever-changing environment, dealing with very sick patients and having to make judgments in a split second, all with the patient's best interests at the forefront. We are patients' advocates when they are awake and asleep. All of this transpires when they are petrified and at their most vulnerable. Our time with them is short but so valuable and must be true quality time. As we keep them warm and cozy, we administer drugs and assist the anesthetist as they drift off to sleep. We are the last face they see and the hand that they hold. Many patients fear they will not wake up, and we are there to allay their fears and assure them all will be well.

They actually wake up with us as well, but are unlikely to remember it. This is such an important role for the nurse. When dealing with children and babies, it is so rewarding to see them sleep peacefully, and then to be there for the safe administering of the anesthetic. When they awaken, they are often confused and disorientated. We stay by their sides to protect and serve.

CHAPTER 2

The Official Job Description of an OR nurse

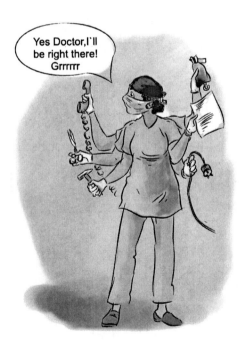

Each OR is staffed with two nurses, depending on the type of hospital and staffing allotments. The surgeons and anesthetists depend entirely on those two nurses to provide everything necessary for their surgery, and believe me, this can amount to lists and lists of specialized equipment, instruments, medications, and solutions—not to mention reams of sutures and stapling equipment. Orthopedics is another story with specialized equipment that is mind-boggling!

Every type of profession has a detailed job description. Behold the job description of the OR nurse!

Secretary: answer two OR phones and various BlackBerries, cell phones, pagers, iPhones, call secretaries, and the emergency department; locate doctors

IT person: troubleshoot monitors and computers for CT scans and X-rays; change paper and ink cartridges

Pseudo-anesthetist: help in all critical situations; watch all machines if anesthesiologist gets called away

Plumber: fix overflowing water or irrigations that run dry while emptying suctions (They slip slide away, as well!)

Electrician: change light bulbs; troubleshoot all electrical equipment when glitches occur

Carpenter: Hammer, screw driver, attach video wires, duct tape anyone?

Photographer: take pictures of unusual cases before, during, and after, videos as well.

Mathematician: count each and every instrument and needle, whether they be huge or microscopic; calculate various drug concoctions

Surgical assistant: assume this role when the regular assistant is busy

Cleaner, porter, garbage collector: all when the assigned people are unavailable

Drug wizard: know all names for all drugs, as well as their locations, how to mix, doses, old names, new names; be able to find them in a computerized drug cart

Gofer: retrieve nitrous tanks, tourniquets, defibrillators (hope not!), monitors, special tables, pneumatic poles, and the ever-elusive pillows

Weightlifter: lift heavy legs or arms; turn patients; move every patient all day after every surgery, despite being "dead" weight (bad term!)

Deejay: many surgeons want specific music played, turned up, and turned down

Contortionist: crawl over cords, under machines, around equipment, and often in the dark (Surgery through a scope is usually done with the lights out for better viewing on the monitor!)

CHAPTER 3

The Two Types of OR Nurses

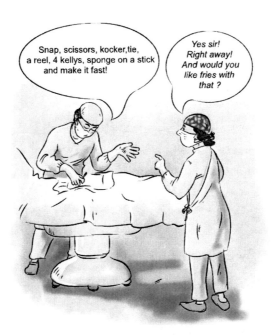

Care always begins with your circulating nurse. The circulating nurse must check the video equipment. She ensures that all the instruments are available and working before surgery begins. She picks the appropriate sutures and staplers for each individual case.

She warms up the bed with a special warmer, as the operating room is often quite cold. She sets up the fluid warmers, suction machines, ART (IV's that go into an artery not a vein) lines, and catheters (to be inserted after the patient is asleep). The pressure pumps are applied to the patient's legs, and the instruments are then counted—yes, we count everything before, during, and after surgery—quite the task at times!

When all the team members are present, we do as airline pilots do and complete our safety checklist. We must calm our terrified patient and listen carefully to the answers as we ask him or her questions. We try to comfort patients as best we can while scanning the chart for all appropriate test results, consents, drugs to be given, blood to be arranged, and so on. At this point, patients are often afraid, and questions upset them further, but it's crucial for the nurses to know they have the correct patient, surgeon, side of the body, procedure…and the list goes on. We also ask about allergies, which is really important! Sometimes this actually annoys people, but we have never met our patients before. We need to know who they are!

Remember also that our nursing licenses are always on the line, and there is no room for error. All our *t*s must be crossed and our *i*s dotted.

Now the circulating nurse rushes over to assist the anesthetist with putting the patient to sleep. This is crucial for the safety of the patient, and most anesthetists will not proceed without a qualified OR nurse assisting. Once the patient is stable, the circulating nurse quickly returns to the "scrub nurse" to pour out all medications, making sure the scrub nurse has sterile labels for everything. This is at precisely the same time when the surgeon needs the CT scan brought up on the computer! The circulating nurse drops everything and completes this task while the mighty phone has probably rung at least four times with multiple questions about the next patient.

Now the surgeon has decided that the patient is not in a good position, so off the nurse runs for pillows, bolsters, head rings, sand bags (heavy!), and tape to hold everything in place. But the tape is gone!

And now it looks like we have the wrong OR bed! The patient needs to be on a slider. Different beds perform different functions—the circulating nurse hurries and searches from room to room before another patient ends up on the bed they need! Some surgeons are very good and help with these tasks.

The difficult part is moving the huge electric bed from one OR to another. Once one is found, the real fun begins! Trying to manipulate a huge, cumbersome bed through congested hallways, tripping over cords and trying to avoid bumping other patients—yes, nurses are furniture movers, too!

Now, our intrepid nurse must turn from technician and furniture mover to Florence Nightingale—all before any instruments are handed—while comforting a sobbing patient.

The scrub nurse is the one who wears an extra sterile gown and gloves. Now, *here* is where we have the person who hands the instruments!

While the circulating nurse is checking equipment and the patient, the scrub nurse sets up all the instruments. This is also a highly skilled job. The instruments are not just "knife, fork, and spoon," as we say in jest. It's complicated, and there are so many of them that often these skilled professionals choose to only work in one specific area so they can really become an expert.

In some countries, there are technicians trained only in a "scrub" position. These individuals are not registered nurses. Many hospitals are employing them as well as Registered Practical Nurses. For Canada, this is a recent practice. It, of course, saves the health care system money.

Orthopedics requires years of experience to master all the tools. These people usually have more mechanical tendency than others and prefer the challenge of the widgets, reamers, drills, and saws. Others prefer delicate cardiac or neurosurgery where patience (and a strong bladder!) is needed, and the instruments are more delicate than orthopedic tools, for example.

Currently, the latest and greatest kind of operation is called "minimally invasive" surgery. This is accomplished through tiny incisions and lots of telescopic lights and cameras. The instruments usually need to be put together and plugged in to various machines and TVs.

CHAPTER 4

Ever Changing

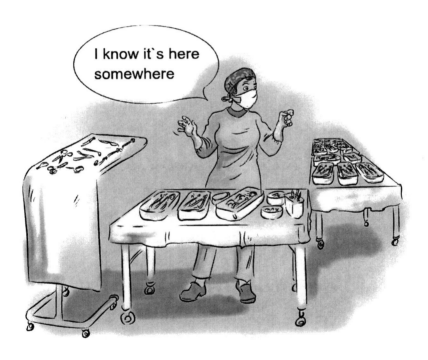

Sometimes, just when your day is organized and all is going smoothly—BAM—an emergency case comes through the door! There are no special rooms waiting for this sort of thing. The OR that is in between cases is chosen to handle the emergency—anything from a ruptured aortic aneurysm to a gunshot to a Caesarean section.

These cases are fit in between one surgery finishing and another starting. The team flies into action for a totally different type of surgery than what they had prepared for. Emergency patients require acute care. For example, they may have just eaten before the event that brought them to our door, and therefore are in danger of aspirating as they are induced for their anesthetics. This is because the stomach contents start to rise and the patient has no gag reflex, so the contents can now slip into the lungs...bad idea. This is where a skilled anesthetic assistant (for example, an OR nurse) is invaluable to saving a patient's life even before the life-saving surgery begins.

On the other side of the coin, the scrub nurse must now totally reorganize herself with different instruments and drugs—all in record time, of course!

Despite the unexpected drama, this calm under pressure is when the OR nurse thrives—it keeps the circulation going! The downside of dealing with emergencies is the problem of now-delayed pre-scheduled surgeries. Pre-scheduled patients take time off work and make many plans in order to work their lives around having a procedure. When an emergency occurs and potentially bumps a patient who has been waiting months, it now becomes a juggling issue for the person in charge of running the OR for the day. Do we ask nurses to stay late? Do we cancel an operation and try to reschedule? How many late rooms do we already have? How many staff members are on the next shift? Lots to plan!

Recently, when this occurred, several nurses had to stay to let other nurses go home as they had young children to attend to. Usually, everyone helps out and steps in to relieve a nurse who cannot stay. This domino effect influences all the emergency cases planned for the evening. You've heard of the little old lady waiting two days for her broken hip to be fixed? This is the reason.

CHAPTER 5

Charting and Passwords

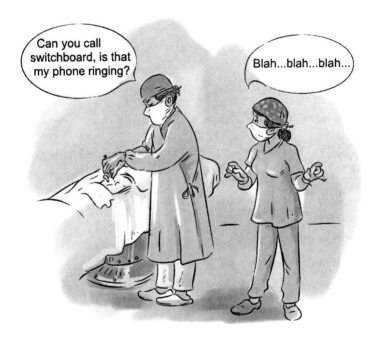

OR nurses must record times for *all* surgeries. This is mandated by the government and also reported to a government body. So it's imperative that it's accurate! (But, eek!—we really don't have time to chart all the times!)

The following times must be filled in on our operative record regardless of whether we have a ten-minute or ten-hour case.

0740 room ready

0742 patient in room

0745 time antibiotic given

0746 anesthetist begins

0753 anesthetic induction

0750 SCD leggings applied

0800 anesthetic ready

0812 procedure start

0830 tourniquet time on (except for a Caesarian section)

0900 urine sent to lab

0905 bed ordered

0915 time baby born (if this is a C section)

0917 placenta delivered

0952 culture taken

1000 x-ray ordered

1025 procedure finished

1028 patient out of room

1030 anesthetic finished

1130 patient discharged from PACU (recovery room) to the floor

If there is a delay, we must record the delay time and reason, which may be the patient arrived late, an outpatient delayed in prep department, or an emergency case came up. This is listed on a separate page.

Don't forget the serial numbers, nurses! All serial numbers on all machines must be recorded, too. All this while being the patient's advocate, charting every movement, and performing all the jobs on our job description list!

The OR is also an ever-evolving world of passwords. It is fraught with them, and of course, they are all different! We have passwords for e-mails, passwords to access patient records, and passwords to access lab results. We have different passwords to access hospital-related education. There are even passwords to acquire all drugs, emergency or otherwise. Some are assigned to us; some we must choose. Most of them expire in three months, and then we are given another. UGH! Who can remember them all? It is never ending!

One day when we are in the nursing home we will all be babbling numbers and letters!

CHAPTER 6

Hazards

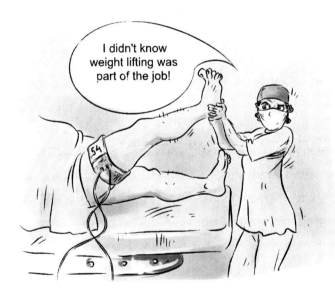

Yes, there are many! The OR comes complete with different hazards than any other area in the hospital.

Objects:

Every day we OR nurses run an obstacle course. Some of the hazards are covert, some obvious. Daily, we climb around, through, under, and over spaghetti-like cords. Our machines have sprawling legs on which to catch us when we run from job to job; there are also buckets to kick and drapes upon which to trip!

Sharps:

There are many sharp objects on which to get cut. These come in a variety of shapes from shiny scalpels (clean or dirty) to needles of every shape (also clean or dirty) to harpoon-size needles (clean or dirty!). When they are dirty, they are *really* dirty. They can be infected with TB, MRSA, HIV/AIDS, VRE, flesh-eating diseases, and more. Very unpleasant indeed! We are ultra-careful to prevent contracting these modern bugs.

Smoke:

The covert danger may be the worst. Every day we breathe in carcinogenic smoke. For many years our different machines billowed smoke when used to stop bleeding in most surgeries. Some of this is just plain smoke, and some is actually burning cancerous tissue! UGH! It wasn't until the last ten years that "smoke evacuators" were used. These machines are still in their infancy but are a step in the right direction. Laser surgery is more prevalent now with many types of lasers. However, all blast smoke.

Gasses:

These are used to keep patients asleep and can be very powerful. We have scavenging systems in place that are quite effective, but there is always risk, especially in pediatrics, as gasses can leak out of the patients' airways—but we won't go into that!

Formalin:

All the tissue to be inspected by a pathologist goes into a solution called formalin (formaldehyde). In many hospitals, an OR nurse pours this over the specimen in an open container. Formalin is known to be highly carcinogenic (cancer causing).

Blood and Mucus:

Yucky but very real. We have the potential to be splattered by both of these flying objects when we least expect it! Hence the shields, masks, and protective goggles we wear…usually.

Flying Instruments:

Think it couldn't happen? Think again! Less now, but it used to occur a lot a few years back!

SARS:

Now that was a hazard we could have done without! During this bleak time, all hospital staff was at risk. The OR was closed to everything except emergency cases, but all staff had to report for work. We were essentially quarantined, and many staff requested to stay home—even without pay. No one wanted the risk of contracting the disease or bringing it home to loved ones, but alas, attendance was compulsory even if you were pregnant.

Those were challenging days, to say the least. We were either farmed out to help in other areas of the hospital because "a nurse is a nurse is a nurse…" (which, as we know by now, isn't necessarily so). Many nurses chose to work screening all people entering the hospital.

This was done at ridiculously early hours in a cold, makeshift corridor. N95 masks had to be worn at all times. These masks allowed precious little air through and often gave people rashes and sores on their faces. We even had a special space suit to wear in the event we had a suspected SARS patient for surgery. It had a little fan inside that was supposed to cool you, but it was extremely claustrophobic.

CHAPTER 7

Rewards

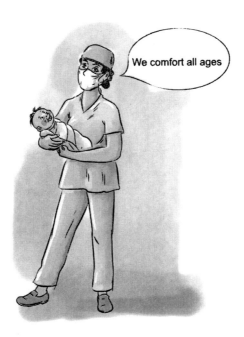

Now for the good news…and there is good news!

The hazards of this job may be many, but the rewards outweigh the obstacles. It all combines to make the job exciting. It is living on the edge every day.

The entire OR staff has a special camaraderie. It starts with the sharing of a lounge area. As mentioned before, OR staff members usually have very little time to eat or take breaks, so we have our own place where almost everyone brings their lunch to sit around a table and chat. If there are nine operating rooms, then maybe three to four people will be there at one time. This also encourages generous people to bring treats! We have to eat at a time convenient to the surgeries and can't always buy food at those hours. This setup really fosters teamwork. Working this way, we all become like family.

CHAPTER 8

Fact or Fiction?
Anecdotes from OR Survivors

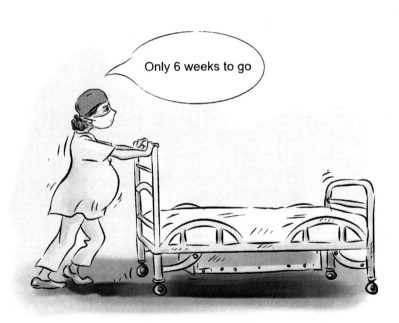

Only 6 weeks to go

Many years ago we had a brand-new surgeon come to our hospital. It was his first night on call, and he had a fractured right hip to fix. Hip surgery involves placing the patient (usually a very old lady—this one was ninety-nine!) on a fracture table. Both legs are suspended and extended and strapped down. One leg is in traction. (Don't ever break your hip!)

After the sweet lady had her spinal anesthetic, she became quite agitated and somehow flipped herself right off the bed…except her feet were strapped in! She was unhurt, and luckily, her head didn't even touch the floor. Everyone was in shock after this, but of course, we picked her up, dusted her off, and carried on. As I plugged the nitrogen cord into the power source, the drill fitting broke and flew across the room, narrowly missing the assembled staff!

With all this stress, the surgeon began sweating profusely and asked me to wipe his brow. Like a good nurse, I did, but I didn't know he wore contact lenses. I wiped them both out!

Needless to say, they were lost forever, and he has never forgotten that day!

**

Emergencies—gotta love 'em!

The operating room was all set up for an emergency (STAT) Caesarean section. The patient was rushed through the doors, and we were ready to start when another surgeon ran in saying, "Stop! I have a ruptured abdominal aneurysm to do STAT!" The patient was taken off the bed, and another surgery was set up for the aneurysm! Most places would not have enough available staff to run two to three operating rooms at night.

Many years ago, in a hospital far far away, a very respected surgeon finished a very difficult resection a part of a patient's bowel. As he removed the large retractor from inside the patient's abdomen, he realized, to his dismay, that he had sewn the bowel around the retractor!! A quick thinking nurse saved the day be suggesting they get a huge pin cutter from orthopedics and just cut the retractor! It worked like a charm.

Then there was the time we had just acquired pneumatic poles. These made it easier to raise large bags of fluid up very high for certain procedures. The problem is, they have a large knob on the side which if you are not careful, it can catch on the tubing running from the very large fluid bag, pulling it out and showering everyone in close proximity with sticky fluid.

**

One day another emergency C-section was all set up with the patient ready to begin. The surgeon came in and said he had another woman whose needs were more urgent also needing a Caesarian, and to take the first patient away. This meant that all instruments and supplies had to be changed, even though they had not touched the patient.(rules regarding sterility)

Guess what? Not two minutes later, another surgeon came along to inform us his patient had just come through emergency, was still fully dressed, and was deemed more needy than the first two patients! Lets dissemble everything and start again! Fast!

What a night!

CHAPTER 9

Personalities

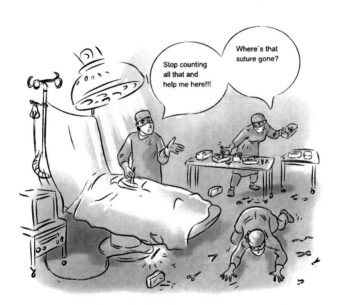

Personalities—wow! We have many!

The Surgeon

- The one who stops everything to talk and talk...
- The one who—push, push—sends for the next patient, but we haven't started this one!
- The one who curses throughout surgery.

- The one who complains about every instrument.
- The one who always blames the instruments for difficulties.
- The one who can use anything you have: "Don't run off. I'll use whatever you have."
- The one who whines, "I've used that for twenty-five years. Why don't you know?"
- The one who always arrives late, then rushes everyone to catch up.
- The one who makes you a secretary—"Answer my phone, call my office!"
- The one who mumbles so you can't hear what they want.
- The one who never remembers nurses' names so calls them all "Sunshine."
- The one who wants you to hand every instrument and also remove it from his hand so he doesn't look away from surgery…and he is very fast!
- The one who sings loudly through surgery (but can't sing).
- The one who stresses all day about being on time and toward the end thanks everyone for being the A team.
- The one who changes glove sizes every week and wonders why you get it wrong.
- The one who can't work with "new" nurses and must be coddled.
- The one who says, "Don't give me what I ask for; give me what I need!"
- The one who says all the time: "Come on, girls, let's go!"
- The one who thinks every job is the nurses'; repair lights, chairs, temperature control.
- The one who always whines "Can I have?"

The Anesthesiologist

- The one who is always late.
- The one who is always on the phone.
- The one who is always on the computer.
- The one who is helpless, messy, and needs a hand with everything.
- The one who needs no help and helps the nurses with everything.
- The one who is neat, neat, neat!
- The one who is always looking for extra work.
- The one who never stops talking.
- The one who says, "Whatever you say, boss," all the time!
- The one who asks the smoker if he or she has read today's paper that says smoking is bad for your health.

The OR Nurse

- The one who is old and "crusty."
- The one who is young and eager.
- The one who is young but always calls in sick.
- The one who is old and deaf (lots of those).
- The one who is always helpful and ready to work.
- The one who is old and set in his or her ways.
- The one who is young and knows it all.
- The one who is always cheery.
- The one who is slow but willing.
- The one who is always around in an emergency.
- The one who claims, "I have never used that equipment before—ever!"

CHAPTER 10

Believe It or Not!

These are all objects we have removed from patients' bodies:

Worms
A Bic pen
Vibrators
Bags of cocaine
A #8 billiard ball
A can of deodorant
A shot glass
A wine bottle
Spice caps
A hand cream tube
A pencil
A champagne flute
A bat (not baseball)
Knives, forks, and spoons
A sewing needle
An eight-inch salami in the wrapper
Safety pins
Plastic bread-bag tabs

Multi-fiber wire, cut and twisted to a knot
Nuts and bolts
A toothpick
A broken dental plate
A carrot
A paperweight
An Old-Spice talcum bottle
A zucchini
A light bulb
A broomstick
Bamboo
A nail-polish bottle
A shampoo bottle
A gold chain and ring
A dildo (homemade)

I will leave the particular orifices to your imagination, but they are not always where you may think!

I am sure other OR staff could add many more when they read this.

CHAPTER 11

The Olden Days

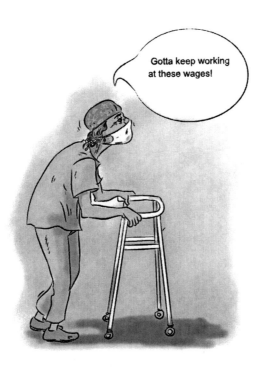

I've worked as a nurse long enough to be able to tell you what it was like before some of our modern conveniences. Here's a glimpse into life in the sixties and seventies.

Nurses wore dresses called "hoovers." Yes, like the vacuum! We wore white stockings, white shoes with cloth covers, and a lab coat when leaving the OR suites. The masks were made of cotton and were reusable. They were washed, rolled up, and at the ready in bins beside the sinks where we scrubbed. The hats were ugly cotton, white, and kind of looked like they belonged to the French Foreign Legion. All hair was tucked in and no jewelry was allowed.

The dresses wrapped around the body, we were absolutely forbidden to wear pant suites/scrubs.

We scrubbed our hands with hard nailbrushes that came in a dispenser you activated with your elbow, and you cleaned your nails with a wooden stick! This scrubbing of hands—up to the elbows—had to be done for ten minutes! No nail polish was ever allowed. The tap was usually accessed with your knee.

The physicians all wore scrub suits and had cloth boot covers that were changed every day and laundered.

The sterile gloves used for surgery were washed, powdered, and autoclaved (in other words, used again and again).

Needles were sharpened, and some were "threaded" by nurses and re-sterilized.

All the sterile drapes, sponges, and tubing of every kind were reused. The drapes were all cloth. It was all very environmentally friendly! Very "green," literally and figuratively!

We had no "super-bugs" back then. Strange, you may think.

SMOKING

Of course, this was done everywhere. Not in the operating room but in the hallways, at the main desk, and throughout the hospital. Lounges billowed smoke!

CHAPTER 12

Present Day

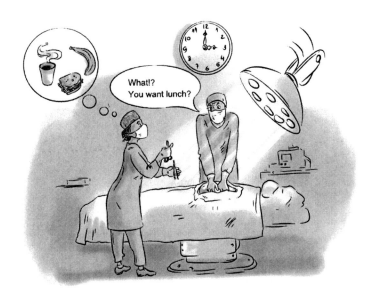

Nurses are permitted to wear scrub suits, not dresses!

All staff members in the operating room wear their own shoes, and no boot covers are required.

Many staff members launder their own clothes and hats, and some even wear them back and forth to the hospital.

<u>Everything is disposable</u>. The masks, hats, all drapes, sutures, sponges, tubing, and so on are used once and then disposed. It all goes into the landfill. As in all things, many changes bring great improvements and some…not so much! We are not very "green," but it looks like there is a push to go back to reusable supplies.

And of course, smoking is not allowed anywhere on hospital property now.

CHAPTER 13

In Praise of Our Ancillary Staff

The operating room could not function without our many behind-the-scenes staff members.

It all begins with the SPD staff (supply, purchasing, and distribution). These skilled workers wash all the instruments, and then assemble, wrap, sterilize, and organize them on carts to be sent to the OR for the next day's surgery (and in many cases, for the present day, as well).

Equally important and indispensable are the people who clean our ORs and transport our patients everywhere. Without them, we could not function. They bring our patients to us with tender loving care, providing them with warm blankets and kind words. They clean the operating rooms after every case and—trust me—this is often a very messy job! Some hospitals have staff that only cleans and staff that only porters. At our hospital, they wear both hats.

There are also respiratory technicians who work closely with the anesthesiologist, especially with the very sick patients. This takes some pressure off the RN (OR nurse).

Surgical assistants are a big part of every hospital. Some are family doctors, some still have practices and some only assist.

Then there are the RNFAs (registered nurse first assistants), who are registered nurses and take a special course in assisting. We love these girls because they also help us, and we tend to be chronically short-staffed!

In our hospital we are in close contact with the pathology/quick-section room and have interaction with their support staff. In cancer cases, we personally deliver pieces of tissue for instant analysis.

X-ray technicians are needed for many procedures throughout the day. They are there to find fractures and kidney stones and to make sure the surgeon is in the correct spot for surgery, perhaps the correct level for back surgery (meaning, between which vertebrae).

Maintenance department is always at our beck and call. Most ORs are extremely busy, and the wear and tear on all machinery is ongoing, so maintaining the machinery is crucial.

This may be a big surprise, but hospitals are under huge budget constraints in Canada. The busy teaching hospitals are awarded more money than the very busy community hospitals. Saving money is always at the forefront of purchases from sutures to microscopes. Everyone endeavors to be mindful of the high cost of doing business in a hospital.

Conclusion

So there you have it—a window into the world of the operating room nurse.

We are the patients' advocates, awake and asleep.

We are the hands, the organizers, the facilitators for our surgeons and anesthesiologists.

We work through the stress of bad times and count ourselves lucky during the good.

And we never lose sight of our ultimate goal: to "carry that lamp" as best we can.

Thank you for sharing in a small piece of our world. I hope you enjoyed this sneak peek into operating room life. Maybe if you come to visit us someday, you will feel more at ease knowing the skilled team is all on your side.

THE BEST TEAM PLAYER I EVER KNEW

A scrub nurse at the sterile field assisting with an operation had run out of curved hemostats.(clamps) The surgeon was using straight hemostats and was unhappy with them. The alert circulating nurse placed another package of curved hemostats quietly on the back table for the scrub nurse to use. The next time the surgeon asked for a hemostat, the scrub nurse gave him a curved one.

The surgeon stopped the operation (you know how they are) and said, "I thought you told me you didn't have any more curved hemostats."

Being the team player she was, and not letting on that the other nurse had given her some, she replied, "I am bending them for you, sir…"

— Author Unknown

CPSIA information can be obtained at www.ICGtesting.com
Printed in the USA
LVOW07s1740160315

430768LV00034B/1691/P